Living

Testimony

Living Testimony

Testimony

By Gwen Peters

A story of divine rescue from **M.S.**,
autoimmune disorders, & demonic affliction.

*"He sent out His word and healed them,
snatching them from the door of death."*
Psalm 107:20

Contents

About the Author

Gwen has been married to her best friend and favorite adventurer Cory for 26 years. Together they love to travel, eat, explore, and visit with friends. They raised three amazing children and two dogs in America and Ireland, and currently reside in the Willamette Valley in Oregon, USA.

Recommendations

"This book will take your breath away. Gwen's journey of healing is nothing short of miraculous. Her honesty is refreshing. And the insight she has learned in the trenches and shares with the reader here is priceless. Testimonies carry an anointing–if you are in need of healing or freedom from bondage, you **NEED** to read this book. God has put it in your hands for a reason; He wants *you* to be free too."

—Holli Aparicio, Minneapolis, MN,
www.allthingsprayer.org

"Gwen's experience with healing and the way she has allowed God to lead her in it has greatly impacted my own journey with healing. The Hebrew word for testimony is 'aydooth', which means "do it again with the same power and authority". Our testimonies are meant to inspire others to have faith and believe that God will do something just as amazing in our own lives. Gwen's story does just that. The way she intertwines scripture with her experiences with God opened my eyes to see His power and authority in ways I never realized before. This is a testimony I will keep handy and read often as I have learned something new from it every time I have read it."

—Jen Miller, Ham Lake, MN

"This is a powerful story of a woman chasing freedom against all odds with only Jesus holding her hand. Gwen generously shares her story in order to see the captives set free and to be obedient to her best friend Jesus at all costs. Her chronicle encourages us to throw away the traditions of man that we may not even know we have, and accept the healing Jesus has for us all. She is a truth seeker and teller, a freedom lover.

If you have felt hopeless and lonely in your journey, you will be greatly encouraged and may even experience healing while reading this. This story helps reiterate the truth that God is ultimately good. What he did for Gwen he wants to do for you. 'Heal the sick, raise the dead, cleanse those who have leprosy, drive out demons. Freely you have received; freely give' "(Matthew 10:8).

—Felicia Hart, Lebanon, OR

Acknowledgements

What began as a desire to share my story with close friends has evolved over a few years to the publishing of the testimony that you now hold in your hands.

Thank you Holli for the initial God-inspired suggestion and second edit of this publication.

Thank you Christy for letting me share my story with you at "1847", and for jumping in for the first edit! I appreciate your openness more than you know.

Brent and Pam, I know you didn't feel like you did much, but your help with general publication knowledge, graphics and media was invaluable to me; thank you so very much.

Thank you Nicole, Shawn, Felicia, and Monica for speaking God's heart into the sails of this venture that I wasn't sure I even wanted to hoist.

Susan, my gratitude to you can never be expressed. Without your courageous, bold testimony, I would be at best handicapped, possibly bedridden, or at worst dead right now. The trajectory of my life and others who read this story will be forever altered because of your faith. You share in this harvest.

To my kids, Dannen, Jocelyn and Gabe, thank you for putting up with me as I learn and grow. Having a zealous mother can be trying at times. You are and always will be my favorite people.

Thanks to my husband Cory who has always supported everything I have ever put my hand and heart to.

Most imperatively, I can never, ever say thank you enough to my Jesus. I never knew You were so good.

Forward

In the fall of 2019 I went to a 4-day conference in Albany, Oregon, hoping to meet with Jesus in a powerful way. On the first evening, a Wednesday, the organizers had an exercise for meeting with the Holy Spirit that I participated in, but I was disappointed because I didn't seem to get anything out of it. I had wanted so badly to have a tangible feeling in my body. People were visibly having a great experience, and I was deflated, feeling nothing.

Thursday was a really good day. We picked up a friend from our church, Kent, because he hadn't yet gotten his driver's license since being healed of blindness in June. When the morning session was done, the teacher asked who in attendance was outgoing and would be willing to have a stranger join them on a "treasure hunt" (purposefully looking for ways to help people meet Jesus). Those willing were invited to the front of the auditorium to be partnered with a more timid individual. Because I am outgoing and wanted to meet someone and take them with me, I went up. A pretty redheaded gal named Gwen came up to me. We prayed and then got together with my husband Kerry and Kent, and went to lunch.

We went to a local diner, thinking that would be a great place to witness and pray for people. As we sat there eating our lunch, Gwen shared her testimony of being healed of Multiple Sclerosis and other diseases. Kerry and I just stared at each other and then conveyed that I also had MS. We were all ears! She had experienced so many healings. It was amazing! By the time we got done hearing her testimony and eating lunch, we all went back to the car. Before we got in, I asked if they would pray over me for healing of MS. I didn't even realize the powerhouses of faith who prayed over me: Kent who was just healed of legal blindness and Gwen who was radically healed of MS and many other issues. So right there in the parking lot, the three of them prayed. I didn't feel any different, but I was full of faith just hearing Gwen's testimony.

That afternoon during the teaching time, the leader said that if anyone went through the exercise the night before and didn't feel they got anything to remember that it planted a seed; that it was there, and it was in God's hands to work with the seed. That evening during the worship time I started to get a slight headache. I sat down and my brain began to feel as though it was being zapped all over by electricity. I asked God what this was, and I heard him say to me, "I am rewiring your brain." "Oh, wow!" I thought. My head felt funny that evening, but I was very excited.

Friday night during worship, it happened again, and although it wasn't as intense, it was definitely happening. I knew I was being healed of **MS**! About a week later I noticed my clarity of thinking was better, I had more control of my emotions and my cognitive issues were significantly improved, including my short-term memory. I was still contending for my eyes to be 100% healed. (Optical neuritis was my very first symptom of **MS**, and it still gave me problems.)

In the course of time, I went to the eye doctor to have an examination and get new glasses, as mine had just broken. Historically, I had never enjoyed eye exams due to my left eye being slower as a result of the **MS**. As I sat in the chair and started to go through the tests, I realized the exam wasn't causing any pain or fatigue in that eye, and it was keeping up with the test. Usually I would have to wait for it to catch up and focus. I started to get pretty giddy inside! I asked the doctor to do all the tests and to really focus on my left eye. She performed all the tests and I almost jumped up and down in my seat! My eye was HEALED; no issues, no fatigue, no pain. I asked her to look at the optic nerve that was damaged and had scar tissue. She obliged me and said the optic nerve was perfectly pink- no scar tissue, no damage seen! YES! PRAISE JESUS! I just kept telling her this was a miracle. On top of that, she said my eye prescription had gone backwards by two years. My new eyes were almost 20/20! Praise God again, as I still happened to have an old pair of glasses from two years ago. This was the confirmation I needed to know that without a doubt, I was healed of MS. To top it off, Jesus was healing the damage left by it. He is so good! I couldn't wait to tell Kerry and the world!

That night, Kerry and I went to an outdoor worship event in Salem, and Gwen unexpectedly met me there. We embraced, and she said, "Can you and Kerry pray for me?" She knew of my faith, and the power of faith displays in miracles! On Sunday at church, I shared my testimony of being healed of MS and how God healed my eye without me even being aware of it. We ended up having an altar call and hi-jacked the rest of the service! Amen. More Lord Jesus! More testimonies of your goodness!

Monica Shaha
Albany, Oregon

Introduction

In the final stages of getting this testimony ready for print, I've been reflecting on how God prepared me to walk this path. As you will read in the following pages I, like many of you, suffered from a young age with dark oppression. I, like many of you, was given very little help in the way of dealing with, let alone understanding, what was happening in my life. And yes, this sadly includes those in the church who seem to have intimate knowledge about God and the Scriptures. Perhaps that is why I was comfortable and felt safe being tutored by Jesus alone in my physical healing journey. I love my spiritual brothers and sisters in the church, but they were little to no help in walking out the victory Jesus paid for me to have in the demonic realm. Jesus Himself had to teach me and lead me into victory. He did this through His living Word (Hebrews 4:12). It was amply tested in the very difficult and lonely journey walking out my freedom from torment.

From this experience, I knew God's Word (the Bible) could be trusted completely. In learning to wield His Words as a sword. I saw the results of doing so prove to be powerful and sufficient in demolishing every evil entity that came against me. And to be honest, looking back I wouldn't have had it any other way. During these trials I felt isolated because of my struggles, but now I have a love relationship with Jesus that could never be taught or fabricated; it's come from years of one-on-one teaching directly from His heart and Word.

Sharing my story is a scary thing for me. There are things that have run so deep in me, that are unspeakably precious; letting it out to the world to possibly be "trampled" causes me to want to hold my pearls of great price close to my heart for safe keeping. But that's not what we are to do with testimonies, because we need to proclaim and hear what God has done and is doing if we are to overcome in this life. My deepest desire in sharing God's story in my life is that you will open yourself up to what He would like to speak to you personally.

This retelling is not about arguing theology. It's not about shaming any one or anything except the devil. It is simply *my story*, how God peeled away the layers to set me free and prove His Gospel true. My story may challenge your long-held understandings, or what you have been taught. God will never offend his Word, but thankfully He will offend our understanding of it if need be.

In this journey I have learned that God doesn't speak just to speak, He always has intent behind His Words, and those Words have the power to carry out His will. By virtue of the fact that you have picked this up and have chosen to engage tells me that God has things he wants to say to you. As you read my story, I encourage you to, with upturned palms, ask the Lord for ears to hear and a heart to learn. Maybe it's time for you to engage with The Healer. He's better than we think He is.

"Bless the Lord, O my soul, and forget not all his benefits; who forgives all your iniquities, who heals all your diseases, who redeems your life from destruction, who crowns you with loving kindness and tender mercies, who satisfies your mouth with good things, so that your youth is renewed like the eagle's." (Psalms 103:2-5 NKJV).

Gwen

1

The Backdrop

I was born and raised in a small town in Oregon. My parents were hard working lower-middle class folks. My mother worked in a hospital billing office. My father, an ordained minister in the Mennonite church, worked in a sawmill. I have five siblings, but for most of my childhood memories it was just my sister Karmin and I, as our family has a gap of seven years between numbers four and five, and I came in at number six. We were latchkey kids from the time I was in first grade. We attended a conservative church very regularly (three times a week in those days) and at age 11, I knew God wanted me to devote my life to the purpose of sharing His love with others. He had a calling on my life that somehow I knew definitively. I didn't understand the How, but knew the What and Why.

When I felt this call on my life, I had begun attending a local Christian school. This was, not coincidentally, when the demonizing began.

I had what I consider a pretty decent growing up experience. I loved my school and my many friends. I excelled in sports, music, and leadership. I had a safe home and always had enough of everything I needed. I had ample opportunity to explore my interests and passions. I wasn't a great student in the classroom, earning average grades, but my extra curricular activities were meaningful and life giving.

I joined a youth ministry organization when I was 19, moving across the country and going full-time as a stateside missionary worker. I met my husband Cory during this time. We married in 1997.

To understand my journey, I feel it is important to go back and share what the years previously held for me. As I look back through the first couple decades of our marriage, I see many things that went under the radar that all eventually came to a head that spring of 2017...

2

The Long Beginning

We were living in Mankato, Minnesota in 2001. We moved there when our first son Dannen was not yet two years old. Cory was working full-time on his four-year degree at Minnesota State University. He worked the overnight shift at the Fairfield Inn and attended classes during the days; I worked part time at the YMCA. We lived in a couple of different places at that time.

We attended an Evangelical Free church in Mankato. This was the time when our pastor's wife, Sue, introduced me to the material from Neil T. Anderson called "Bondage Breaker". Anderson taught about spiritual warfare, something I had been engaged in already for 15 years, but never had anyone who could remotely speak into my experience the way his teaching did. It began in sixth grade, after several dark experiences babysitting at strangers' houses and witnessing bizarre things through demon-possessed girl who attended my Christian school.

When I say "spiritual warfare", what I mean is that dark spirits taunted me almost every night. I would endure "small things" like being startled or scared by an evil presence just as I drifted off to sleep by something moving in the corner of my room or something flying in front of my face, to dark smothering dreams, sleep paralysis, and evil manipulations of voices and things in my room.

I remember coming to a point when my daughter Jocelyn was just a few weeks old, with a knowing if I did not break the cycle of torment I had experienced almost every night since I was a pre-teen, my kids would be the next target. I remember seeing myself in my mind's eye in a doorway, knowing I had to step into freedom in this area for the sake of my children, but being terrified and motionless. How I knew there was more, that there was freedom to be had, can only be explained as a "knowing" from God. People didn't talk about this kind of stuff. My faithful church-going friends and family didn't understand it, so the most response I ever got was an, "I'm sorry," a glassy-eyed, "I'll pray for you," or a track handed to me.

So when I came to this breaking point, I knew God was the only one I could turn to. That day stays fixed in my memory, as I managed through shaky tears, "Lord, you are going to have to move my feet." And He so faithfully did. He sent my then pastor's wife, Sue, to me to get me started. Thus began my first major journey of learning about my authority and identity in Jesus, which eventually bled into my journey with health issues.

This was the first time I remember noticing things being a little off physically. One day I noticed that my eyes saw colors slightly differently; one side saw more blue while the other saw more green. I was intrigued by it, but didn't give it too much thought. After Jocelyn's birth, I didn't start my monthly cycles like normal. I knew it could take a while to get things going again; and although I wasn't breastfeeding, I thought little of it. We had begun taking a natural birthing class around this time, as we wanted to utilize this practice moving forward in our family planning. I had begun taking my temperature daily, and logging it in my class notebook, when it became apparent I never quite got into a given temperature range. I was pretty happy about it, thinking how nice it would be to not have a monthly cycle. But then I mentioned it to my doctor, and he decided to look into it further. I went to the clinic and had my first ever MRI. It revealed an issue with my pituitary gland. So they started me on a medication that cost $76 per month. I thought that was a huge rip-off. I eventually stopped taking it (mostly because we couldn't afford it), but my cycle started again, so I didn't give it more headspace.

I began having severe pain in my right side at certain times. One time when we had just had a delightful evening at an Italian restaurant in Minneapolis with our friends, Pete and Roxanne, I had an attack on our way home. They drove me to the ER, and after many tests, the doctor did not have a definitive answer for what had caused it. After more tests and following up with my GP, it was determined I had gallstones. The gallbladder secretes liquid to help digest fatty foods. My doctor said because of the size of the stones, they would just have to take my gallbladder out. Not being presented with any other options, I agreed, and they removed my gallbladder. I remember this being difficult because Cory had to take time away from his busy schedule to stay home while I was in the hospital. We relied heavily on friends because we had no family in the area to help.

Our children were little, and Cory was working 60 hours a week and taking 17 credits his senior year of university. I remember the strain of this time. The kids were about five months and two and a half years old, when I contracted strep throat. My friend Nedra came over and took the kids for a few hours for me because Cory had to work. But there was nothing else to be done, so I just soldiered on. This became my mantra, although I never voiced it as such. But you get good at pushing through when you have no other options.

3

The Trudge

The kids and I moved to Oregon and lived with my parents while Cory went to Virginia to take an unpaid internship at an airline, with hopes of landing a job there when the internship was completed. I took a job working at a local grocery store in the customer service center. I decided to start cosmetology school during this time to help the family out with a second income.

In 2003 we moved back to Mankato. I finished up my schooling. Then in 2004 Cory got a job with his first airline, and we just kept soldiering on. We would have the same day off together about once per month. The kids were five and three. During that time I contracted walking pneumonia, but we weren't allowed to miss school, so I just kept on. My friend Colleen watched the kids for "peanuts" during the day when I was at school. It was during this time that

I got pregnant with our third child. After I graduated, I got a job working part time in the evenings at JC Penney Salon, and driving a school bus in the mornings and afternoons, toting the kids along with me.

I don't remember a whole lot during that time, just that there was no resting. I was in practicality single parenting most of the time, and working the two jobs. I enjoyed my work at the salon, but finding childcare was always a chore, so I would trade haircuts and colors on the weekends for childcare, as we didn't have the cash for it. We also gave plasma for grocery money, which we were grateful for, because the plasma center actually provided childcare. I never gave any thought to what my body was saying, because it would have been futile. I simply didn't have the time to.

We bought a house, and after my youngest son Gabe was born in 2005, I developed a hernia on my left side, and needed surgery to repair it. During those months I remember having a few emotional moments, although I never let it slow me down. I kept soldiering on. I gave up the bus driving and went to work at an insurance agency during the day. Cory was working three jobs at that point; life was hard.

His family was going through some really rough times. One day he came to me in tears and said he didn't know what to do. He said he was ready to throw in the towel with his career, one that we had felt from the beginning was ordained by God. As we cried out in fatigue and confusion, we prayed and asked God for a rescue.

The next day that rescue came. A captain with whom Cory flew at Mesaba Airlines told us that an airline based out of Ireland was looking for crew to help transition a fleet of planes they were acquiring from Mesaba, and wondered if Cory would like to go. It took us all of three minutes to decide that we most definitely did want this change. We felt like we hit the jackpot, or were being led to the Promised Land. He would be able to work only one job, and I would be able to stay home with the kids! So we packed up the house, found renters, and headed to Ireland for what we thought would be a yearlong adventure.

4

New Cultures, New Battles

Our time in Ireland lasted longer than a year. Cory was enjoying making a livable wage for the first time, and I was thrilled to be an at-home mother full time. We could think of nothing better.

After we had been there a little more than a year, I noticed that my tongue was swelling up huge. My tongue had never fit well in my mouth, always resting between my bite, so I brushed it off. I was getting frequent cysts around my ears, and had recurrent mouth ulcers. I remember showing my oldest child, Dannen, my tongue and he remarked, "Whoa, mom!" But then the swelling would go down off and on. I had started researching essential oils, and I began incorporating these into our lives (this was before Young Living and doTerra were around). And I just kept soldiering on.

Jocelyn got stung by a hive of hornets around this time; we counted about 30 stings. I look back now and see that this was the beginning of a devastating downward spiral for her.

Gabe had always been a bit feisty. Retrospectively, I can see how his first years were pretty traumatic. He was very angry most of the time, but especially in the mornings when he would wake up. We were often at a loss to know how best to parent this precious little guy. I remember standing in church one morning and crying out to the Lord about him, saying, "If he behaves this way until he's 18 years old and out of the house, I will still praise you." We were singing, "You give and take away, You give and take away, my heart will choose to say, Lord blessed be Your Name," and as clear as if He had said it audibly to me, the Lord said, "I will return to you the years the locusts have stolen." I dropped to my chair, in instant sobs, and grabbed my Bible, because I remembered these words were somewhere in there! I found them in Joel 2. I interpreted His words as that He was now giving where He had taken before (but I look back now and know He was correcting my theology - He was definitely giving).

From that time forward, Gabe woke up with a smile on his face and a laugh on his lips in the mornings.

I had heard of a homeopathic practitioner from some friends, so I took us all to see him. We had a number of things that needed attention, so we began dishing out money to see him. His methods were successful in many ways, and we continued to see him as needed over a few years.

My slight little Jocelyn, however, never stopped having things to deal with. It was as if we'd fix one thing, and another would pop up. So after reading a book on preparing foods like the ancient peoples did, I started doing things like converting to as much organic and whole foods as I could, soaking grains, and taking long shopping trips that were hours away to get the food I felt we needed to heal us and keep us well.

In the fall of 2010, Jocelyn stopped growing and got even thinner than she already was. I thought maybe she had a tapeworm. So I ended up taking her to the clinic, and with a simple finger prick they were able to diagnose her with Type 1 Diabetes. We both left the clinic in tears, and after a quick stop at home to get a change of clothes and toiletries, and to take the boys to our friends house, we made our way to the Temple Hospital in Dublin for what ended up being a week long stay and to learn about life with diabetes.

5

I Need a New God; This One

Doesn't Work

This story isn't about Jocelyn specifically, but I need to mention it because something changed in me then. I felt like God had abandoned me, that He could do something, but that He wouldn't. So it was up to me to try to take care of my family. I was teaching Sunday School, I was homeschooling my kids, and I was doing a pretty good job at it. I still believed in God, I still taught my kids about Him, I still loved him, but I just didn't trust Him anymore. I had always been an avid reader of my Bible, but I stopped being able to ingest anything I was reading. I didn't realize it, but I was so ANGRY at God. I believed He could've stopped all that had happened, but had just turned a blind eye.

Cory was working six days away, with only two at home between times, so getting up with my sick ten-year-old twice a night for months checking blood sugar levels, counting meal carbs, calculating and administering insulin, checking in with the doctor daily, and revamping our lives in a foreign country with a socialized medical system was completely on me. I steeled my heart, and decided since Cory couldn't help, and God wouldn't, it was up to me.

I had been sleep deprived for years, because of the decade's-long battle with the unseen unclean spirit realm. I felt even then that God was just a silent observer, like a wrestling referee who would just make sure that things didn't get too out of hand; I believed that even though He could stop the torment, He chose not to. I suppose over the years I filled my "why" with religious jargon such as "He's allowing this to make me stronger," or "I need to be humbled," or something like that. So this new life with Jocelyn was just an extension of what I had already believed for most of my life. My parents didn't know about the demonic oppression (I was too afraid to tell them, and having grown up in conservative circles, it was something so out of their experience that they did not know how to help when I did tell them). When we got married, Cory didn't know how to help, and was extremely taken up with school and job responsibilities, so he also wasn't available to me. This new thing with Jocelyn was just more of the same message: **YOU ARE ON YOUR OWN.** So I just kept soldiering on...

One night I remember jumping out of bed, because I felt like a bug had crawled into my left ear. I could feel the tingly, crawly tickling down in the cavity. I went and got some oil to drown it out. I worked at it for probably 1/2 hour. In the end, nothing came out of my ear; I was perplexed and had no answers.

Another time, I developed a rash on my left breast. I was taking homeopathic care for it, and it did eventually go away. The practitioner said anytime a rash came and worked its way out, it was a good thing. So I rejoiced in my supposed victory, and went deeper into the religion of health and wellness. My dependence on natural knowledge and my own understanding was growing roots. I became emboldened in my new found "salvation".

6

The Extended Vacation

Quagmire

Time passed, and things with Cory's work were changing. After months of prayer and contemplation, and an interview with Emirates Airlines in Dubai, we decided to take a severance package from his current employer, with the promise of a job and a move to Dubai within a few months. We packed up everything, and in June of 2012 we went back to the United States for a summer of traveling with the kids. We bought a van and a pop-up camper, and toured around, seeing 17 different states. During this time we visited friends as we traveled. At a two-week stop over in Arizona, I was talking with my friend Alicia, and broke down regarding my fears about Jocelyn (who had recently needed glasses; I was afraid she would go blind as Cory's mother and uncle were both blind) and Gabe (who also was showing some weird physical signs of something wrong). I see now that my reaction was unnatural, that my weeping was more than fear-based emotion. She went and talked with her husband Nathan about our interaction. In the past Nathan had shown unusual discernment, and he told her, "Something else is going on." I asked Alicia what he meant, and she didn't know exactly, but I remembered his words.

We wrapped up our trip at Yellowstone National Park. We all really enjoyed it. After being at a particularly smelly sulfuric spring, the kids were practically gagging, but I couldn't smell it. They were shocked that I couldn't smell it, but I was mildly amused thinking, "Ha ha, lucky me."

Things with Cory's potential job had stalled, so we were forced to make arrangements for temporary housing and school that fall for the kids. After a few frustrating weeks of online academy, and an emotional breakdown by me, we put them in a local private school. I look back now and am not even sure what filled my time except driving around trying to get my laundry done cheaply. The brain fog was dense, and my energy depleted. I caught a cold at some point, as did Dannen. We both had ringing ears for a few days; his went away, mine never did.

That early winter both the younger two kids were sick with some long-winded bug or parasite, as was I. We went to stay at my parent's house. Floods were making it hard to know if we could even remain at our temporary house (which was a built-over chicken coop), and Cory had to take a month-long contract overseas because we were running out of savings waiting for the job in Dubai to come through. He couldn't draw unemployment; we had a letter stating he'd been hired, we were just waiting for a date for him to start. One midnight I was tending to Jocelyn during this sickness, as her blood sugar levels would not come down. We didn't have a diabetic care team in the States because we weren't planning on staying here, so I felt on my own to care for her. The insulin syringe was acting so funny, so I tried another. The second one was acting very odd too, and that's when the Lord prompted me that it was not a physical thing causing the resistance, so I prayed, and then the syringe started working correctly and I was able to administer her insulin.

About that time I went to the Urgent Care for what I thought might have been strep throat. I told the doctor that I had ringing in my ears. He attributed it to stress. While looking in my nose he noticed inflammation. My turbinates were pretty large, so he referred me to an ENT. They took images of my head, and noticed a large benign tumor in my left nasal cavity. They also performed surgery on my turbinates to help open up my airways. After the procedure they sent me to get an MRI to see if there was anything more sinister going on. I received a call back from them within a couple weeks telling me that there was no cancer.

Spring rolled around, and I was in pretty bad shape. I was taking homeopathic remedies like candy and constantly sucking down herbal medicinal teas; I had stopped eating gluten, and had developed environmental allergies. We went to Disneyworld. I was exhausted, suffering from shortness of breath (I tried Jocelyn's inhaler; it didn't work), racing heart, internal trembling of my extremities, and depression (at DisneyWord, how dumb is that?). While there I ended up in the Urgent Care, where the doctor felt around and found my lymph nodes were inflamed. Because of this along with my trembling legs, he encouraged me to follow up with my primary care physician when I got home. A couple days later I made Cory take me to the ER in the middle of the night for shortness of breath and trembly legs that wouldn't calm. They took a CT scan and declared nothing life threatening was going on, and advised me to see my PCP when I got home.

7

Hell Descending

Very shortly after we returned, I went into a dark hole. I couldn't function. I was on the couch, rocking myself at times. My energy was gone. I felt comatose. For someone who was always in control, who was active and very capable, this terrified me, which only exacerbated what I was experiencing. My body was completely out of control, and I didn't know what to do about it. I was having a true mental and physical breakdown. Cory canceled his plans to do another much needed month contract away, even though our money was gone, and I was whisked off to my sister Karmin's house in Nevada to convalesce. On the airplane, I remember sitting slack in my chair, looking at my toes and thinking how oddly intriguing it was because they were spotty purple.

I had a dream that my family was in a park; we were walking along, and I had to sit down on a wooden park bench because I didn't have the strength to go on. They didn't stop though; they just kept walking, leaving me behind. My sister, who represented the medical field in my mind (she was a hospice nurse), stood nearby looking at me, and I remember screaming in extreme fright to her, "Sister, don't leave me!"

While I was lying in bed one morning at Karmin's house, I was listening to music. A song by Kari Jobe came on. It's called "Healer". When a particular line of the song soon played, it was as if the Lord turned the volume way up, and I heard, "You walk with me through fire. You heal all my disease." I didn't know it fully then, but that was a stake in the ground in my journey. That phrase lodged itself in my spirit.

During this time, we got a call from Cory's folks who told us his 40-year-old, non-smoking, marathon-running brother had been diagnosed with lung cancer. His prognosis was not good.

Not long after this we got an email from Emirates Airlines that they had had a delay in their aircraft deliveries, that they were dumping the current pilot pool. The job we had been hanging on for no longer existed. That day my left ear made a loud pop. The tinnitus worsened. We sunk in the mire even further.

I went to a neurologist who did more scans. He showed me some spots in my brain that could be Multiple Sclerosis, or could just be from falling/activity. Having been a very active, athletic youth, it was entirely plausible that it was indeed from falls so I told myself it was nothing.

I remember singing a song in church during that time, and the lyrics were, "Your love never fails, it never gives up, it never runs out on me." I never realized it until many years later, but I always subconsciously mis-sang it as, "Your love never fails... it never holds out on me." Interesting, because that is exactly how I felt about God, that He was holding out on me.

8

The Valley Of Shadows

We moved houses and went from a mouse-infested chicken coop to a mold-infested doublewide trailer, but we thought it was a palace compared to our previous abode. We were elated to have the space and be so close to the kids' school. The two younger kids continued to have health issues, allergies, etc. Jocelyn and I were involved in a rear-end collision. I found a local chiropractor, and we started going to him for help.

After the kids and I started seeing this chiropractor, we had discovered some structural issues with both the boys, and he began working on them. Jocelyn and I just didn't seem to heal, however. We saw him for two years. The insurance company thought we were stringing them along, but we were sincerely not healing. My left shoulder had continual pain; I chalked it up to the school bus driving I was doing as a job. And I soldiered on.

We switched to an office of Osteopathic Doctors to try to help us. During this time we were having 2-4 medical appointments every week, between all of us. We were taking hundreds of dollars worth of nutritional supplements. We did have some success with these. It didn't fix things, just seemed to delay most things; however, we kept going to these doctors, spending thousands of dollars every year.

I noticed one night in the middle of the night that my eyes were doing funny things. I had finished looking at my cell phone in the dark, and then when I put the phone away, I could barely see out of my left eye. If I kept my left eye closed, it would happen in my right as well, but my left was definitely the worst. I went to the eye doctor who ran all sorts of tests. She was researching on the web about what it could be, and I prompted her to just say what she was suspecting. She responded that it could be **MS**, but it was a really random thing, and she couldn't say definitively. She put me through a battery of in depth tests that all came back inconclusive, showing no abnormalities. I just chalked it up as interesting, but that was it. And I soldiered on.

I started coaching volleyball, and since I loved the game so much, I thought it would be a good outlet. At one point I must have landed on my bottom during practice. I thought I had gotten a spider bite; it turned out to be a huge cyst on my backside. It got so bad and big that it went into my bloodstream. I ran a fever and started feeling ill, so I was put on antibiotics and had it lanced. During the first round of antibiotics, I had a severe pain in my left arm. It hurt so much, I was wondering if I was having a heart attack. So I took myself to the ER. No heart attack; they just deemed it a random event. The first round of antibiotics didn't work, however, and I had to have a second one. It took months for the cyst to heal.

In the fall of 2016, I noticed pain in my left arm even more. I started to get numbness in my left foot and my left fingers and arm. Additionally I was starting to choke on my own saliva. That was weird and seemingly random. It was always comical for my family, because I have this unique characteristic that if I choke on something, like a crumb down the wrong "pipe", I cough and then sneeze, *always* - usually a few times. They all gather 'round and say, "wait for it... wait for it..." and then I'd sneeze, and they'd whoop and holler and congratulate me. We got to and "celebrate" a lot those days.

My stamina had plummeted; the anxiety had returned. We went to a friend's house in Las Vegas, those same friends we had visited years ago in Arizona. On the way down we stopped at a rest area. By the time we got to their house, I figured I had accidentally touched some sort of fungus and had transferred it to my eyes, because I had these red sores under my eyes that to me looked like ringworm. While we were there, Alicia told me about our mutual friend Susan, who had been healed of a dairy allergy. She suggested I go and talk with her. I filed it away as the shadows continued to swallow me.

9

A Guttural Hearts Cry

After the Christmas break that year, I went back to the Osteopathic doctor. She had told me earlier that fall that if I ever had trouble with one side of my body, to let her know; she explained it would indicate MS and that my brain was not communicating with one side of my body well. She obviously had her suspicions. This time I had a check up, and she encouraged me to go get another MRI, because I still had the tinnitus as well as hearing loss, and she was concerned about the symptoms I was experiencing. She also put me on a trial run of medication for my thyroid that she had tested and had come up wanting.

We went on a family ski holiday. I didn't enjoy it. My circulation wasn't working well, and I was getting numbness in many places. That made it hard to ski. I was very sensitive to the cold. I was anxious. And after a few days on the slopes, my left thigh started hurting pretty badly and was tingly and painful. I had just started taking omega 3 fish oil, so I assumed the reason I was feeling all the tingly sensations was because things were healing.

A week or so later I got a call from the nurse to ask about the MRI I had had a few years back. She questioned me and said, "They told you everything was okay?!" I replied in the affirmative. She said, "Because the doctor looked at the scan and it's evident you have [a condition where the lining of your nerves have been eaten away]." I thanked her for the phone call and decided I wasn't going back for another MRI. She said the doctor wanted me to read a book on treating Multiple Sclerosis and other autoimmune issues with food. I said I would do that, and I did.

I bought the book, and I devoured it, so to speak. I believed this to be God's answer for me. He was going to heal me through food! So I figured out a plan and began to work the plan. After a week I did start to notice a difference with my eyesight. But three weeks in, although I was seeing some results, I started to realize how unsustainable this was (nine cups of veggies per day?!), how much it was costing, and how much time it was taking away from my family. This was supposed to become my new lifestyle, and this was God's answer? This didn't feel like deliverance; *it felt like bondage.*

The kids were still in private school at this point, and I had more free time to myself during the days than I had probably ever had in our married life. I was exercising (or trying to) one day, and I remember my left leg shaking so badly, I couldn't hold the stretch. And I broke. I just broke. I knew I was losing the battle. I knew I was dying a slow death.

I cried through heavy, desperate tears, "Jesus, help me!"

10

"What if it's true?"

Susan was walking past my house one day, and she had just finished asking the Lord who she should give a certain Bible-based devotional book. As she walked by my driveway, the Lord told her to give it to me. She felt a little awkward about that, since we'd barely spoken in 20 years, but she went with it. She went home and gave me a call, giving me a brief testimony of her healing, and invited me to tea at her house if I wanted to come.

Alicia had already told me she had been healed of her dairy allergy. I honestly had never heard of anyone who had been healed supernaturally of something like that, so because I was intrigued, I went. She was my neighbor, after all. We had moved out of the double-wide a year earlier, in part to get away from the mold and dust (allergies) in the valley. She was now just a half mile up the road!

We had a nice visit. I asked her about her healing. Susan had a round worm and parasites years ago that wreaked havoc on her body, along with yeast, allergies, and other autoimmune issues. She told me briefly about it, and how she came to believe her healing was already paid for by Jesus, and how she was able to receive her healing. She wrote the name of a teaching on a yellow Post-It note and gave it to me. It said, "God Wants You Well".

I went home and told Cory about our conversation. I sat at our counter on a bar stool a little stunned and asked him straight out, "What if it's true?" He shrugged, we sat in silence for a bit, then he left to go about his day, while I sat there thinking some more. I made a decision and proposed to myself, "I'm not about to be hoodwinked." So I grabbed my Bible and went to the computer. I put my Bible out in front of me like a shield, and said, "Holy Spirit, you promised you would help me and guide me into all truth (John 16:13 NKJV). Don't let me be led into some weirdo false religion." With my Bible in hand, I looked up the teaching on the Internet. Attached to the teaching was a video of a healing testimony. I clicked on that testimony to watch it, not knowing what it would be about.

Remarkably, it was the story of a lady who had been healed of *Multiple Sclerosis.*

11

Desperate Gulps of Living

Water

Th**is** began a concentrated time of searching, reading, listening, studying, and following as the Lord began to open my eyes to His will through the Scriptures: that He indeed wanted me well, and that He had provided the way for me to be well.

That same night after my conversation with Susan, I went to bed. I was barely awake when I felt that familiar tremble in my legs, so I murmured experimentally, "In Jesus' Name, legs be still." And they obeyed.

From my journal: *The next day I decided to stop following the food-plan and go back to just my regular gluten-free eating. God showed me that following the special diet was for me a plan B, in case God didn't heal me. But that's not faith AT ALL. I want God and God alone to get the glory for my healing. If I'm going to be consumed by anything, I want it to be the Word of God. I'd rather spend my time learning God's truth about healing than being consumed by what I'm "supposed" to eat, always wondering what I'll eat next. I cannot minister to my family or others when all I can manage is about food, trying to attain healing, when all along Christ has already purchased my healing through the atonement.*

"Now the Spirit expressly says that in latter times some will depart from the faith, giving heed to deceiving spirits and doctrines of demons, speaking lies in hypocrisy, having their own conscience seared with a hot iron... commanding to abstain from foods which God created to be received with thanksgiving by those who believe and know the truth. For every creature of God is good, and nothing is to be refused if it is received with thanksgiving" (1 Timothy 4:1-5 NKJV).

I continued to watch testimonies of people who had experienced healing and study the Word about what it had to say about healing. I bought a Greek and Hebrew concordance, and began dissecting and searching. In my heart I truly did want to believe, but there was still a catch in my spirit. I didn't understand it, but I knew there was hesitation when I said, "I believe."

12

The Chain That Held The

Elephant Fast

I went and took a shower and cried out to the Lord for help, for faith. He then showed me what was stopping the flow of healing. He said, "You have a spirit of abandonment." I stood there shell-shocked; I knew that word was bang-on. I began to sob, knowing he had put his finger on a key to the shackles I still wore. You'll remember I talked about the belief that God could do anything but wouldn't? I realized that that stemmed from feeling abandoned (emotionally) by men in my life and ultimately by God himself. I saw in an instant that through the decades of demonizing that started as a pre-teen, along with other emotional upheavals in my life, and culminating when Jocelyn had been diagnosed with diabetes; I accepted the lie that I had been abandoned. I even recalled a time 15 years earlier when someone did some investigating on me to discover that at one year old, I had accepted/experienced emotional abandonment by my dad. (This would have been during a terrible, traumatic time in his life as well.)

I did not realize I was the proverbial elephant that had been chained by a small stake as a baby. But at this point in time truth uprooted that lie and, after most of my life, I was walking away. I renounced that spirit; I declared I was done with it, that I was not abandoned and had never been, and I was indeed free at that very moment.

Being free from a lie is something many have limited understanding about. I learned a few things from this key event that I took forward with me into the journey of walking about my healing. I had believed for years that "getting free" was a monstrous battle, and this mind set kept me in a place of perpetual exhaustion. It was as if I had to be on alert at all times. I saw that this was actually a working of my flesh because in my heart I didn't trust that God would help me, that I had to keep probing and digging, not realizing that all this really did was keep me distracted by focusing on my enemy, and not focusing on my Savior.

I also realized that freedom could happen instantly because Jesus already did the heavy lifting. This was a new concept to me, as my previous teachers (experience, peers, and biblically illiterate adults) did not understand this concept. Scripture tells me He broke every chain (past tense) (Psalm 68:18-19; Colossian 2:15). There is nothing left for Him to do; He did all that is needed, and sat down at God's right hand in finality (Hebrews 10;12-14) to watch His victory play out. In Ephesians 6:10-20 I'm instructed once about "wrestling" and four times about "standing". The battle isn't in trying to get free. The battle is to stand in freedom, to keep the ground already taken. This battle is in our minds, which must be renewed according to the truth of God's word. While modern philosophy (that most of the time does not even consider the re-born spiritual part of our being, or has a darkened understanding of it) may tell you it will take months, even years, to be free of past trauma, addiction, or pain, Jesus says differently. Look at His life! While the Word implanted in our souls will often be tested, it's not because freedom is hard to come by; it's the lie that we are not free that has to be put to death. And I was empowered to see this victory in real time in my body and soul.

13

Sick and Tired of being Sick and Tired

A paradigm shift was happening. I was realizing I not only had the option of getting really mad at sickness, I had the mandate. I had lived with disease for so long, it got into my brain (mindset, thinking). When one has thought "sick" for so long, it goes unnoticed how comfortable and familiar it becomes. When I zoomed out for a panorama, I realized there are whole subcultures built around sickness, communities to belong to around these curses that come against us. Disorder becomes "homey", and sickness can actually be enjoyable, especially if one has failed to fit in or feel accepted in other ways. As twisted as it sounds, I had become that person, sick in my body and mind.

I saw I desperately needed the Lord to help me see sickness as he does. In this journey I have experienced that often breakthroughs didn't come until I or another person just got fed up with our state of being. This would most often come after a time of prayer. I know that is the place where I came to, where I was desperate enough to let God back into that area in which years ago I'd years ago shut him out. The years gone, the money spent, the time invested, in trying to deal with illness - I was like the biblical account of the woman with the issue of blood, who spent all she had on doctors, and only grew worse (Luke 8:43).

The day following that huge revelation in the shower, my eye was doing a thing I had been experiencing for months, a stupid twitching, fluttering thing. I was walking through the Costco parking lot, and I got so mad I firmly told it to stop in Jesus Name.... and within a minute, it did! There was still a slight eyelid movement, so I resolutely said again, "Eye, I told you to be still." And after a bit, it was. Additionally, that day my outside left foot was numb, so I cashed in my shared Jesus-inheritance (Ephesians 3:6), declared healing over it, and it went away.

"Therefore submit to God. Resist the devil and he will flee from you" (James 4:7). This says that God doesn't cause the devil to flee. It's our job to resist him by submitting to God, and then telling the devil where he can get off - but he doesn't flee until we resist in some way. Not that it's a huge battle; it's just a position of authority. Additionally, after years and years of failed flailing's around this issue with the demonic realm, I have found that a brief spoken stance (Ephesians 6:10-18), followed by audible worship of our amazing God, is one of the most powerful weapons against the enemy. It's almost comical how fast the enemy flees when we lift our voice in praise to Jesus, entering into God's presence and light! I love this. It never gets old.

As I was so new on this path, I began to feel anxious and have doubts. I cried out to the Lord and opened my Bible. According to my journal, these verses were waiting for me at first glance as I did:

"O LORD my God, I cried to you for help, and you restored my health. You brought me up from the grave, O LORD. You kept me from falling into the pit of death... I cried out to you, O LORD. I begged the Lord for mercy, saying, "What will you gain if I die, if I sink into the grave? Can my dust praise you? Can it tell of your faithfulness?.. You have turned my mourning into joyful dancing. You have taken away my clothes of mourning and clothed me with joy, that I might sing praises to you and not be silent. O LORD my God, I will give you thanks forever," (Psalm 32:2, 8-9, 11-12 NLT).

14

Who Will I Listen To?

Who's voice do I listen to? Do I submit to God's words? Or do I submit to my doubts, to religious jargon, or to the natural ways of thinking through a carnal mindset?

"For to be carnally minded is death, but to be spiritually minded is life and peace. So then, those who are in the flesh cannot please God" (Romans 8:6-7 NKJV).

Oh how I wanted to please God with my mind, and I knew I must continue to root out old, death-ridden ways of thinking.

I wrote verses and truths on my mirror, on my phone lock screen; I put sticky notes up all over the house, on the dash of my car, anywhere my eyes would rest. I wrote the promises He'd shown me in the Scriptures and plastered my living space with these life-giving living words (Hebrew 4:12) to keep my mind focused on those truths. I played Spirit-filled, God-centered worship music constantly. I stopped searching for answers to symptoms and illnesses on the internet. Thank God I didn't have social media at that time either. I hunkered down in a sense. I instinctively knew God was doing some major gardening, pulling up old, harmful beliefs and planting His Word (Mark 4). Those seeds were precious, tender, fresh; I did not consult with many at this time about what He was teaching me, my primary teaching was from the Word and the Lord. Under His guidance, I protected those seedlings.

There are so many voices that get in our face if we let them. With the increase of social media, news sources, limitless information on the internet, and media influencers, it really does take a great deal of effort to shut out all the noise. God's voice is real and able to be deciphered, but we have to be willing to shut out all the other sounds and focus on Him.

One morning I was getting ready to go back to my osteopath. I was supposed to be getting my "long term" thyroid dosage that day. I suspected God didn't want me strapped with a disease. But could I be healed instantly? I stood by my refrigerator in my kitchen and said, "Thyroid, be healed in Jesus' Name." Then I went to the appointment. When I got there, and they got me checked in, the doctor came in and tested my thyroid. She said, "Ope! Guess we don't need any medication anymore. Your thyroid is perfect." I wanted to jump out of the chair and shout!

I became *convinced* God wanted me well, and he kept confirming it to me through the Scriptures.

15

The Blame Game

I'd been taught that "nothing happens to us that isn't God's will", and "we just can't know the mind of God..."; comforting words that there is some higher purpose for His "abuse". I believed, therefore, that all of the twisted, cursed things that came against us were all God's doing, at least indirectly. I began to see Him as this abusive celestial parent, who would physically hurt a person (or let his hit man Satan do it and take the fall) just so the person would have to depend on Him more, or because the rebellious person hadn't learned their lesson about something and needed to be humbled more. So resembling a wicked game, like the movie Misery, He'd break my ankles for his own, mysterious, higher purposes. To be holy, therefore, I must "suffer well" under his hand, right?

But... if I believed it was God's will for me to be sick or infirm, why didn't I just lean into it, go all the way, really please God by just lying there and taking it? Why did I seek healing from other methods? *Would this not be hypocrisy?* If I was being intellectually honest, I would have stopped going to doctors and stopped taking "all the things" to cure myself, because I would be actively rebelling against Him in seeking health or a cure. I really would have just waited mutely and submissively, strapped willingly down to the table, and thanked Him for shattering my ankles, because He surely knew best.

Specific passages of Scripture began to come to mind, and were helpful to me as I wrestled with the beliefs I had always taken for granted, but was now questioning.

"The thief does not come except to steal, kill, and to destroy. I [Jesus] have come that they may have life, and have it more abundantly" (John 10:10).

"But the people did not receive [Jesus]...And when his disciples James and John saw it, they said, 'Lord, do you want us to tell fire to come down from heaven and consume them?' But He turned and rebuked them, and said, 'You do not know what manner of spirit you are of. For the

Son of Man did not come to destroy men's lives but to **save them' (Luke 9:53-56)." (**Greek: sozo; it means "deliver, protect, heal, preserve, save, do well, be/make whole.)

"But as it is written: 'Eye has not seen, nor ear heard, nor have entered into the heart of man the things which God has prepared for those who love Him.' But God has revealed *them* to us through His Spirit. For the Spirit searches all things, yes, the deep things of God. For what man knows the things of a man except the spirit of the man which is in him? Even so no one knows the things of God except the Spirit of God. Now we have received, not the spirit of the world, but the Spirit who is from God, that we might know the things that have been freely given to us by God. These things we also speak, not in words which man's wisdom teaches but which the Holy Spirit teaches, comparing spiritual things with spiritual. But the natural man does not receive the things of the Spirit of God, for they are foolishness to him; nor can he know *them,* because they are spiritually discerned. But he who is spiritual judges all things, yet he himself is *rightly* judged by no one. For 'who has known the mind of the Lord that he may instruct

Him?' *But we have the mind of Christ*" (1 Corinthians 2:9-16, emphasis mine).

One morning I was meditating on the Bible passage in Isaiah 54, particularly where it says, "by His stripes we are healed", and Jesus asked me quite abruptly, "They didn't torture the animals that were sacrificed in the Old Covenant, so why did they beat me?" It stopped me in my tracks.

I remembered a discussion a relative was having with my mom about the 24 hours leading up to the crucifixion of Jesus. This person was upset, and really just calling out God about the brutality of it all. She was verbally wagging her finger at Him, saying, "It didn't need to be so gruesome and violent, " and essentially, "shame on Him for letting it go that far; it was senseless and poorly thought out". I also remember my sister and I being shocked at her arrogance, "You would criticize God Almighty on the way He planned out and fulfilled the most critical event that has ever happened in the history of the world?!" We were indignant... but I never understood the why of the brutality, *until this moment.*

"Surely He has borne our *griefs and carried our *sorrows...But [Jesus] was wounded for our transgression, He was bruised for our iniquities; the chastisement for our peace was upon Him, and by His stripes we are healed" (Isaiah 53:4-5). (*In the Greek, "grief" is the word "choliy", which means malady, anxiety, calamity, disease, grief; the word "sorrows" is "makob", which means affliction, pain, sorrow; "stripes" means a "weal", a physical black and blue mark, hurt, wound.)

Jesus Himself interprets the Isaiah passage for us. "When evening had come, they brought to [Jesus] many who were demon-possessed. *And He cast out the spirits with a word, and healed all who were sick, that it might be fulfilled, which was spoken by Isaiah the prophet, saying: 'He himself took our infirmities and bore our sicknesses*" (Matthew 8:16-17, emphasis mine).

16

Unintended Consequences

To be well I realized I needed to be healed in my gut, as so many maladies including brain diseases are connected in the core of our being. I was standing in my kitchen one day as I thought over these things. So just as I did with my thyroid, I told my digestive system to be healed. I began eating gluten immediately, believing God healed me, and to this day I have had no issues with gluten.

A by-product of having my gut healed was something that didn't even enter my mind. You see, for as long as I can remember, I had been allergic to alcohol. When I was a kid, we didn't have alcohol in the house, but we did have cough syrup that had alcohol in it. When I would take the cough syrup I would IMMEDIATELY have to go to the bathroom as my body tried to eliminate it immediately. As an adult, my husband thought I would get used to it and simply start to like alcohol. So every couple years he would come up with something and say, "Oh, try this. You'll like it." But every time, I wouldn't like it. Even when I wanted to like it, I'd get two ounces in and be lying on the table, sick, crampy and woozy and wanting nothing more than to be in bed asleep. I don't remember when it was exactly later that year when I tried some alcohol, but my husband watched me drink 12 ounces of hard cider, and experience zero adverse effects. Amusingly, I believe this was when he became convinced that the healing was real.

At this time I ditched ALL of the hundreds (perhaps thousands) of dollars of nutritional supplements in my medicine cabinet. For me, those were an idol, they were my "plan B". I had for so very long relied on other things to heal me: oils, homeopath, organic food prepared correctly, supplements, etc. In my heart I knew that I must forsake that god completely and swiftly, or *I would never be free.*

I had tried all the things the natural world says to do, but they had never produced lasting results. In my spirit a silent vow was taken. God would heal me, or I would die. I was "betting the ranch". It was all or nothing. No turning back. No plan B. No compromise.

17

Who is Responsible for this

Mess?

A really large component to all of this was understanding the laws of authority as laid out in scripture. God gave the earth to man to care for (Genesis 1:26-28). Man abdicated his authority to the devil, bringing on the Curse. But the law that God bound himself to prevented Him working outside of the authority He set up; He charged man to take care of the earth. Creation became warped and chaotic, because mankind was warped. That's why Jesus had to come as a man, so that He could redeem mankind, take up that authority that was given by God and wield it as a man. When He paid the price for mankind's freedom, and became the Curse (Galatians 3:13), He was legally able to give man his rightful authority back; but He did one better, and gave him God's spirit to indwell and empower him. His blood speaks a better word (Hebrews 12:24)!

I finally came to understand all those years of demonizing were not because God wouldn't do anything to help. As I stated earlier, He already did everything I needed at the cross. But I had to learn my authority because He had delegated it to ME. Again, in the Bible the Apostle James says we must submit to God, resist the devil, and he will flee. Jesus fulfilled all I need for victory; I limited God by not using my delegated authority, which stemmed from not believing that what He said about my authority was true. I had to "press charges" at times and stand up for what Jesus paid for me to have. I was getting bolder, and was determined that Jesus paid way too high a price for me not to get what was mine through his finished work. I saw clearly now that to settle for less was to *dishonor his sacrifice.*

A fire had been ignited in my spirit. All of these truths were mounting and I was indignant at the loss I had suffered, and so sad for the destruction my family endured. I was furious that my ignorance caused me to be easy prey for the enemy. I became hell-bent on reclaiming all that had been lost.

With my new understanding, my patience with sickness was obliterated. The day came when I realized that those sores under my eyes were eczema. So I told those nasty things to go. The next morning, they were gone. However, when I went to get my youngest son Gabe out of bed, what should be on his face but eczema! Time to press charges. My ire immediately rose up. "Ooooooh, no you don't!" So I rebuked that eczema on him. It went away, and the next morning, guess what was back on my face? So I commanded it to be gone again, and to not attach to another person again.

This opened my eyes even wider to the battle we were in, and it wasn't against flesh and blood.

18

I Have No Idea How to Do This

I was driving one day to Albany to take a course on home health care to become a practitioner for a job, ironically, for that first chiropractor that treated us after our car accident. I was listening to a healing teaching on the way there. In this testimony, the teacher was saying he was praying over a young man who was blind in one eye. He prayed and prayed. Nothing was happening. He dismissed the group they were with, and he continued to pray. After about half an hour the Lord said, "He doesn't need healing, he needs a miracle." The teacher asked God, "What's the difference?" At that same time the other minister who was there said, "God just told me He doesn't need healing, he needs a miracle." So the teacher said, "What happened to your eye, son?" And the young man proceeded to tell him that when he was a baby he got an infection, so they took part of his eye out." Bing - the light went on. So the teacher commanded that previously removed part to come into his eye, and within a few seconds the boy could see perfectly out of that eye.

I pondered this throughout my training session, and on the way home as I was driving down Seven Mile Lane, I thought, "If I'm going to have a healthy digestion, I need to have a gallbladder. My brain needs digested fat to be healthy." So I determined in myself that when I got home, I was going to call a prayer line and have them pray with me for a new gallbladder. Immediately the Holy Spirit said, "What do they have that you don't have?" I was chagrined, and thought, "uh......", coming up blank. So not really knowing if I was "doing it right", but knowing God just told me I had what I needed, I said, "In Jesus Name, gallbladder come into my body." Within a few seconds I felt this little balloon-like thing inflating up under my right ribs. I just about drove off the road. I started giggling and nearly hyperventilating. I didn't even know where my gallbladder was located exactly. So I pulled over, and googled on my phone where the gallbladder is. And wouldn't you know it, it was right where I felt that little balloon sensation up under my rib.

I could not wait to get home to share this with my family. I sat them all down and told them all. I remember the men were mildly interested, albeit skeptical. But not Jocelyn. I had been praying that God would ready her to receive her healing, and as I looked over at her she began to shake and weep. I knew it was a God-moment, and said, "Jocelyn, are you ready to be healed?" And she nodded tearfully, wordlessly. So we went into her room and shut the door. I said, "In Jesus Name, all autoimmune diseases be gone. " At this she felt her nose and head instantly clear up. Her lungs filled with air as the asthma left her body. I said, "Pancreas, be healed." She felt her pancreas grow warm (who ever feels their pancreas?!), although we didn't really know where it was specifically located.

We were both weeping and laughing as she told me what had happened, so we googled that too, just to make sure it was her pancreas she felt. She had a pain in her back, so she rolled over and I laid my hand on her back and commanded it to be healed, and the pain left. She also had a round donut-shaped spot in her belly where there was abnormal internal scar tissue from an injection site - that disappeared.

(As a side note, my kids were all involved in this healing journey, and at the end I'll list all that was healed, but they have their own testimonies to share. I will include them when it ties in with principles I was learning in my story.)

19

Jesus = God's Will in the Flesh

I could no longer doubt that God wanted me well because of the obvious mission Jesus was on which included healing. Hebrews 1:3 tells me Jesus is the exact representation of the Father. God's heart was shown in how Jesus lived his life. As I read and reread the Gospels (the books of Matthew, Mark, Luke and John in the Bible) I learned more and more about how Jesus administered healing.

Now that I had a new gallbladder, I knew I was on track and on my way. My brain had been starved of fat for so many years. I was so excited that my digestive track was healed and whole and was going to start producing life in my body the way God designed it to.

"And he said to her, 'Daughter, your faith has made you *well. Go in peace, and be healed of your affliction" (Mark 5:24). (*sozo, which means "save, deliver, make whole, heal, preserve, do well".)

I was lying in bed one afternoon napping, and those blasted eye twitches had returned. (I think sometimes God uses my groggy times to speak to me cuz I'm still enough then to listen - I love this.) But I rebuked them again, and they left, and I said, "Lord, it's not sticking. What am I missing?" And he said immediately, "brain lesions". My eyes momentarily flew open wide as saucers, but I had been freed from fear, and I wasn't going back, so my thoughts moved forward. I knew what I had heard, and I knew that when He speaks, His words are never flat or two-dimensional. His words have intent behind them; His words are His command, so after only missing a split second, I spoke to those brain lesions, and I knew in that moment I was healed of Multiple Sclerosis.

20

Keep Going!

I have come to understand that God's healing is not mysterious, willy-nilly, up to His "whims". God uses laws to govern the physical realm, and He also uses laws to govern the spirit realm. There is much to learn, and I have by no means got the market cornered, but I am learning more about these principles and how to cooperate with them in order to see His kingdom come here on earth as it is in heaven. I would tell myself often, "Gwen, don't let what you don't know keep you from what you do know." If I don't understand something, I no longer chalk it up to God being his "unpredictable self", or that I can't know His mind and will; we can ask God to reveal to us what we don't understand. He wants to show us himself, so we can be confident we have been granted what we asked of Him (1 John 5:14-15).

When you have wasting disease, it spreads, destroying as it goes. There were so many things in my body that had been touched by Multiple Sclerosis. But I believed fully that not only did God want me healed, he wanted me whole. In the half a year that followed, I just would occasionally uncover something that remained as a symptom of the diseases. I termed these things "lying symptoms", because God had healed me, so those old things my body was holding to were a lie, and needed to completely pass away. But I had a responsibility in this process – I needed to use my words and refute those lies when they reared their head so I didn't entertain any doubt in my mind. Jesus charged us with this responsibility, and gave us His authority to carry out his will (Mark 16:15-20; Matthew 28:18-20, Luke 9:1), so I would speak to these cling-ons with that knowledge, and continued to see things being healed in my physical body.

For instance, that leg that was bothering me after skiing? It didn't clear up on its own. The nerves had been damaged. The root cause had been dealt with already, but the damage was still there. So I had to pray and speak over that.

I learned to seek the Lord on things that weren't lining up with His will as laid out in

Scripture in my body. He was **ALWAYS** faithful to show me. I stopped being afraid that He would show me something scary; I stopped being afraid of having my past understanding challenged; I learned to trust Him again, and perhaps for the first time felt that tangible, consuming love that the Bible tells us He has for us. I began to trust His Word over what my eyes saw, what well-meaning religious teachers would say, even what my body would say.

I looked in the mirror one day and noticed I had these two brown bumps that were forming on my face, raised, near my nose. I thought to myself, "Those are from cells gone rogue." So I spoke and said looking at my face in the mirror, "All cellular malfunction on my skin be healed in Jesus' Name." A couple days later I noticed they were gone. Sweet! But that's not all. You see, I had said "on my skin", not just "skin on my face". Our skin covers our entire body. Back when Jocelyn was a baby, I had a scar removed from my upper left back (it was under my bra strap and was painful, an old zit that hardened over). A keloid scar formed over that area when the doctor removed it, a big one with a black hair that grew out of the center of it, with dark lines where the sutures had been. Not long after the bumps on my face went away, I noticed that the keloid on my back had completely healed and there was no longer that large, squishy raised lump there. It was flush with the rest of my skin. Additionally, I had a nasty spot on my back that had a waxy, bumpy scab, about the size of a large lima bean. I had picked it off a few times before, but underneath it remained a festering wound, so it would scab back over and remain painful and itchy. After this skin-event, I picked at it, and the skin underneath was healed! I got excited and for a few days picked and picked at it, more than I should have, but I was so excited to have the beautiful new skin underneath! It was more signs of health, that my body had ceased to be a weapon against me, and was healing as God had intended in his wonderful creation.

21

What's in a Word?

When God created this world and the heavens, He did so with His words. We were made in His image. He showed me that my words carry power because His words carry power. He says with our words we confess who he is (Romans 10:9), we renounce sins (James 5:16), we speak to "mountains" (Mark 11:23), we refute judgments that are raised against us (Isaiah 54:17), we possess the power of life and death (Proverbs 18:21), and will be held accountable for our words, careless or otherwise (Matthew 12:36). The Bible is filled with examples of blessings and curses that are spoken. I used to dismiss all of this as nonsensical psycho babble, because the first one I ever heard who mentioned this principle was Oprah, and I had long since dismissed her as one without any godly wisdom. But I missed the principle, which is one that can be confirmed over and over in scripture. When we speak in alignment *with His will and in faith*, we can know that we have His power to see His will carried out with our words.

I also learned that things that don't naturally speak audibly could still speak. Yes, we know the story of Balaam's donkey (Numbers 22:28). But there was also the time when the fig tree spoke to Jesus. By the color of the leaves, it was saying it had fruit on it, and a passerby would think there was fruit on it; but it did not really have fruit. It was a lie, a perversion; Jesus answered its hypocrisy by cursing it to death, silencing its hypocrisy. The tree shriveled up beginning at its roots, and the next day showed the results of Jesus' words (Mark 11:20). I realized by this example that my body also talks to me, or rather can lie to me.

That summer Gabe had a Boy Scout camping event. It was hot, and he was not dealing well with it. I remembered back four or five years before that, when he had a heat stroke at an airshow. This was the second time in a couple years for him. He also suffered from cold sensitivity. It dawned on me that his body's thermostat was broken. So I pulled him aside and prayed over him, something like, "Thank you Jesus, for giving Gabe healing. Body temperature regulator thing, be healed." I didn't know the scientific name for what was going on, but that didn't matter. And I sent him back to join his scout troop. He has never had another issue with heat stroke.

Shortly after that I was putting a few pieces of the puzzle together and realized Jocelyn, Gabe and I were dealing with broken endocrine systems. I was sitting on my bed that night, and was unsure if I could just pray over them without them being in the room, whether it would still be effective if they weren't present.

Jesus tells us the story of the Roman centurion who went to Him for healing for his sick servant; this man understood authority, so much so that he said he didn't need Jesus to come to his house, but just asked Him to say the words and it would be done. Jesus marveled to the crowd who was witnessing this that this man had more faith than anyone He had ever seen in all of Israel (Mathew 8:5-13).

As I thought about these things, I figured God was the one who put those pieces together for me, so I just moved forward again, and prayed and spoke over all of our endocrine systems. I noticed the next day that a couple of my lingering symptoms had gone. That was also the day that Jocelyn felt a pain in her pancreas (again, who feels their pancreas?), but that is a story for another day.

I remember praying over my dad one day for gout in his thumb. After I got done, he looked at his thumb, frowned, and showed me, as if to say, 'Nothing happened." I said, remembering the fig tree, "Just wait, you will see in the morning." That night I was lying in bed and almost asleep when it felt like a bolt of lightning shot through my left arm. I cried out in pain, and after the shock of it, I started grinning, and would have laughed if it hadn't hurt so bad. I knew at that point my dad had been healed.

I knew that these were signs that we had hit an area the enemy had his hand on. The demons very often would "pitch a fit" when I'd pray over something. It got to be comical, although it used to terrify me. This concept wasn't new to me. When I started to walk out freedom from fear of demons and their torment about a decade before this, I often saw an uprising in activity, as they were trying to bully me back into bondage, lie to me that I was not really free. They would switch tactics and go after my family. They would get loud and blustery. This type of overt reaction would have sent me into a black hole of fear in my earlier life, where fear had literally been my bedfellow for most of my journey, because night time was when the enemy would come to steal my sleep with demonic activity. But I saw now that the enemy only had control over me when I gave in to him, believed his lies, and forgot my place in Christ, seated and resting in Him (Ephesians 2:6). And I wasn't about to yield that ground again.

Knowing my authority and learning to use my words to partner with Jesus was a complete game changer.

22

Different Symptoms, Same

Cure

That fall I was outside looking at a part of our property with Cory. We were making plans for when my parents were to move up with us. I had this cough and could feel it settling in my chest. I knew I was developing walking pneumonia again, I was recognizing the signs. The chunks I would cough up were thick and green. I also knew God would take care of it for me. So I prayed over my lungs, and told the infection that Jesus said it had to go. While I did continue to cough for the next couple weeks, the mucus was no longer green, but thin and clear. I knew the infection was gone, and just rejoiced as my body got rid of that excess gunk. As a side note, later that winter my Osteopathic doctor was feeling around my chest and asked me if I had recently had pneumonia. I kind of grinned and replied, "Yeah."

My answer was always the same for every issue that came up. The Name of Jesus cannot be trumped (Philippians 2:9-10, Ephesians 1:21-22), it's bigger than any diagnoses and ailment known or unknown to man.

In December of that same year (2017), all areas of my body that had been ravaged had not been restored yet. Much had, but not all. So I continued to seek God on this, never budging on the belief that He wanted me whole, not just healed. One day I was sitting on my bed, and I was seeking Him further about healing. He reminded me of when I had strep throat, and also in that winter of 2012 when I may have also had undiagnosed mono. At any rate, I knew the EBV (Epstein Barr Syndrome) could be a result of those infections. My cousin had contracted that, so I was aware of some of the effects. I felt I should rebuke that virus and syndrome in my body, and command healing over my central nervous system. After that the tingling in my right foot went away, and the extreme pulsing in my ears vacated.

I was caught so unawares when Jocelyn was diagnosed with diabetes, that in the ensuing years

I became expectant and desirous of medical diagnoses. Like many people, going to the Internet and finding out what was wrong with my kids or me or loved ones was a pastime. But what I didn't realize, perhaps as a way of coping, was that I was very quick to agree with those predictions. We are counseled to do just that, after all. Embrace the diagnoses, accept it, get used to it, and work with it. But after more and more labels were put on, I grew weary of them. They soured and gave off a nasty stench of death to me.

It was miraculous to me, then, that through Jesus I was able to have my mind changed. In the past if God would have told me to pray over a certain diagnosis, I would have been terrified. But realizing it was not an issue for Jesus, it became not an issue for me.

23

To Eat or Not to Eat

We had many, many victories in 2017-2018. It was a battle to continue on at times, to not give up at "good enough", or stop believing for full manifestation. I would get tired of standing so long for the manifestations of what I knew God wanted for us. When I would get so tired, I had three "crazy friends" with whom God had connected me, believing believers, to whom I could go who knew how to pray, battle, and stand strong in the spirit, and who would lift up my arms like Aaron and Hur did with Moses when the battle got long (Exodus 17:12). They have helped us see great victories through their extended faith. From my journal I see that He spoke to me during this time to encourage me that this season would not go on forever, that there would be an end to the battle raging over us.

In the winter of 2018, I was visiting a used bookstore with Gabe, and a book jumped off the shelf into my cart. Okay, not really, but it might as well have. I saw the book and knew it was for me from the Lord. It was a short read on the biblical discipline of fasting. This was an area I knew very little about. I took it home, and after reading the whole thing in one go, decided I would begin that night to fast from all food. It was one of the hardest things I've ever done. The enemy tried to attack my sleep the second night, so I knew it was having an effect. I was encouraged to keep going! My goal was three days.

I have not been a person who "pictures things". I don't even use "words" when I'm thinking or have an inner dialogue, like a lot of people do. I think in concepts and ideas. But they rarely if ever had materialized as a visual in my mind. Anyway, during this fast I was taking a bath (I'm convinced my bathroom is holy ground). As I was praying I got a "video" in my head of me walking along this brick road. Up ahead was a castle, and underneath me were these blue, writhing little creatures. They were reaching up from the cobblestones to trip and grab me, but as I walked along, these stones were being set in wet cement and then instantly dried, creating pavement as I moved forward towards the castle. The little demons were being permanently covered over and sealed. By this I knew that my days of torment from unclean spirits were over. Had I never been on this healing journey, I may never have learned of my authority, and thereby always struggled with the menacing little imps. This is huge in my heart. After decades, I was completely free. This will NEVER get old.

I have since learned that a three-day fast will break most strongholds. Fasting does not move God, it changes us by pushing down the voice of our "flesh" and unlocks things in our spirits that allows what God has already provided to be accessed by faith and flow into our lives and spirits, fine-tuning our ears to his voice.

24

Harvest and Replanting

A couple years ago, I was at my hairdresser's. I have naturally coarse, dry hair. When I started to go to her in 2016, she was astounded at just how dry my hair was. In fact she said she didn't know anyone with such dry hair. ("Great", I resigned. My hair has always been a source of contention in my mind as it's been wild and unruly since I was a toddler and even a general source of conversation in my circles!) I get a customized conditioning cocktail treatment every time I go. Well, it was about two years after my initial healing, and I was in for a routine appointment. After she got done with my hair she said, "Gwen, your hair is so happy!" Shocked, I replied, "What?!" No one had ever said such things about my wild head of hair. And then I started doing the math. Hair grows about 1/2" per month, my hair was about to the middle of my back (the longest I'd ever had it, it would usually break off by then). I realized that all the dead, unhealthy, "dry bones" hair had grown out and been cut off, and what was left was the hair that had been growing since I'd been healed. Now that is pretty cool.

In February of 2019, I developed a chain of five large cysts on my lower torso. While I had struggled with cysts in the past, it was only one or two that would come at a time. So I was really frustrated about this sudden blast. I went to Susan's house one day so she could pray with me about it. As we prayed, she sensed the root cause of the cysts was *fear*. When she mentioned it to me, it agreed instantly with my spirit, and I began to weep. A few weeks before, we had found out that our best friends, Nathan & Alicia, had experienced an affair in their marriage. In just another week Cory and I were supposed to go to a marriage weekend conference. I knew I was not just afraid, I was terrified that what had happened with our friends could also be what would happen with us. We had gone through a couple years of not-very-happy marital companionship, so fear was definitely something I was experiencing, but had not faced it. She anointed me with oil and we prayed, and I released that terror to the Lord. The cysts went away in short order, we went to the conference, had a marvelous time, and God assuaged all my fears.

Recently I had some old symptoms try to creep back up. I know I have been healed, so there was no putting up with it. But they persisted, so I contacted my "crazy friends", and had them pray. The symptoms not only stopped, but the lingering trembling legs were restored finally to wholeness! Wow! That felt amazing. A month or so later, the trembling legs did not return, but the other symptoms did try to. After a few days, I was lying in bed, talking with the Lord about this. The verse from 1 Thessalonians 5:23 had come into my mind as I was conversing with him. "Now may the God of peace Himself sanctify you completely; and may your whole spirit, soul and body be preserved blameless at the coming of our Lord Jesus Christ." I said, "Lord, I want to present my body to you blameless, how can I do that when it's acting like it is", and he said, "Your body is rebelling; rebellion is as the sin of witchcraft"(1 Samuel 15:23). My eyes shot open wide and my spirit immediately rose up indignant, and I said, "Heck, no, body. You will NOT be a party to witchcraft. You will stop that this instant!" And the symptoms packed their bags and fled.

I continued to have nervous system symptoms; although the root of **MS** had dried up, the damage left in my body has taken time for me to receive healing over. I continued to stand in faith for complete healing, to be made whole (sozo). In 2019, I was at a conference (the same one where I met Monica, whom you met in the forward of this booklet). We were practicing hearing the Lord. A young man whom I didn't know but sat next to me prayed over me; he shared with me what he saw. He said he saw "MS" come up, but it whooshed away, and then the words "Central Nervous System" came and stayed in his mind. So he prayed over me that day and I was healed of that old symptom.

Conclusion

This testimony was years in the making. My journey through the darkness was filled with many twists and turns, but God in His faithfulness brought me out of the darkness into his marvelous light (1 Peter 2:9). I not only have a healed body and a healed mind, but also a healed relationship with my Heavenly Father.

My children are mostly grown, and as my husband Cory, and I look back we are in awe of how God has met us and helped us get to this place we find ourselves in. Our road was not perfect, seamless, smooth, or without misunderstanding and mistakes. But God is FAITHFUL to make good on all He says when we press in to Him for help. He is faithful to fill in the gaps of our understanding and enlighten His words to our spirits.

I'm learning constantly and do not claim to have complete understanding or revelation on the things I wrote about. Even in the time it took to compile this manuscript for publishing I've learned more from Him about healing as he walks with me through life. I love getting to know Him and hearing daily from Him as he reveals more of himself to me. We cannot exhaust Him, there will always be more of Him to love and enjoy.

These pages are a faithful narrative of the things I have experienced in my life, the things I have learned, the things God has spoken to me. I apply to the witness of God first and foremost, and also my husband, family, friends Susan, Naphtali, Michelle, and Alicia, who have walked this road with me. Additionally, I have my body as a *living testimony*! I could have had a very different story. My desire is that this testimony can be used as a mighty weapon in our hands, that the sword of infirmity the enemy used on me, we can all in turn seize it and thrust it back into him, using what he meant for evil for good and God's glory, destroying His works (1 John 3:8). This is why Jesus came!

If you find yourself harassed by the enemy, assaulted by illness, or plagued with doubt, I want to encourage you that the same God who helped me overcome the evil one's schemes wants to help *you.* He loves you with a never-ending love and he will not give up on you. Run to him with all you are worth and he will meet you and help you and teach you, just like He did for me.

God isn't into formulas. You aren't a puzzle to be solved, you are a treasured child whom He wants to meet with and speak to intimately, heart to heart. He has principles laid out in the Bible, but the most important thing to know is that Jesus is the Healer, and that He wants you healed, made whole and delivered. Nothing in the universe can stop what He's given to us if we are willing to cooperate with Him, and listen to Him above all.

In Hebrew the word *testimony* is "aydooth", which means, "Do it again with the same power and authority." *We overcome by the blood of the Lamb (Jesus) and the word of our testimony* (Revelations 12:11).

Do you need healing? *What God has done for me, He will do for you too. He's better than we think he is.*

Epilogue

For transparency, I wanted to list the areas we (my family) have experienced healing at the time of publishing, and those we have yet to see come about. This is not to "brag" except in Christ (2 Corinthians 10:1). His power is immeasurable, His grace abundant, His work accomplished on the cross complete, and His goodness towards us reaches to the sky.

Full healing manifestations: thyroids, migraines, light sensitivity, brain fog, asthma, eczema, under-weight/failure to thrive, numbness/pain in arms/hands/feet, gut flora, allergies to cheese and other foods/additives, mold, dust and pollen, eye twitching, delayed eye color distortion, cysts, gluten sensitivity, digestive system, pancreas, yeast infections, gallbladder, brain lesions (Multiple Sclerosis), pneumonia, demonic voices/oppression, despair, short legs grown out, endocrine systems, lymphatic system, jaws set in right alignment, gout, flu, colds, central nervous system, nerve sensitivity in the face and ears, random swelling spots on the body, rashes, muscle weakness in extremities, post-covid lung damage, pre cancer cells gone, and mange on our dog. Partial/ongoing manifestations: tinnitus, sense of smell, diabetes.

Made in the USA
Columbia, SC
04 November 2023